Your Pregnancy diary

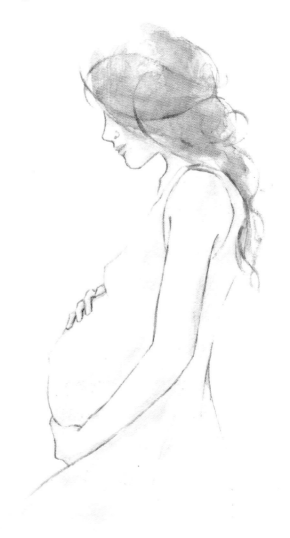

Publishers ~ Howard W. Fisher, Helen V. Fisher
Managing Editor ~ Sarah Trotta
Book production ~ Randy Schultz
Interior design ~ Maricel Albertyn
Illustrations ~ Maricel Albertyn
Cover design and illustration ~ Maricel Albertyn

Published by
Fisher Books, LLC
5225 W. Massingale Rd.
Tucson, Arizona 85743-8416
(520) 744-6110
www.fisherbooks.com

Printed and bound by Tien Wah Press, Singapore
10 9 8 7 6 5 4 3 2 1

Library of Congress Cataloging-in-Publication Data
Nicolson, Tilla.
    Your pregnancy diary : a day-by-day record of your pregnancy / Tilla Nicolson.
        p. cm.
    Previously published: Cape Town, South Africa : Tafelberg Publishers Limited, 1999.
    Includes index.
    ISBN 1-55561-288-1 (hardcover)
    1. Pregnancy—Popular works. I. Title.
    RG525 .N525 2000
    618.2'4—dc21   00-032163

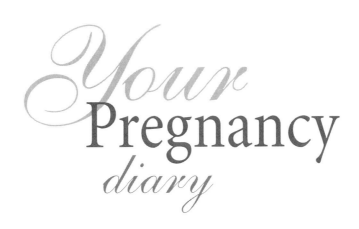

Your Pregnancy *diary*

A day-by-day record
of your pregnancy

Dr. Tilla Nicolson

Illustrations by Maricel Albertyn

FISHER
BOOKS

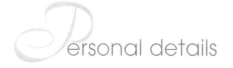ersonal details

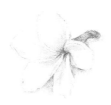

My name: ....

Social Security number: ....

Address: ....

Telephone: ....

Age: ....

Weight: ....

Blood group: ....

Rhesus factor (Rh): ....

Partner's name: ....

Partner's work address: ....

Doctor's name: ....

Doctor's address: ....

Doctor's telephone number: ....

Doctor's partner: ....

Emergency number: ....

Hospital or birth center name: ....

   Telephone: ....

Ambulance: ....

Taxi service: ....

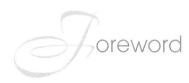

Foreword

This pregnancy diary follows the generally accepted time divisions used in medical science.

The duration of a pregnancy is 40 weeks (or 280 days on average) from the first day of the last normal menstruation. Conception takes place only during ovulation; that is, 2 weeks after the first day of the last normal menstruation.

The pregnancy is calculated in completed weeks; for example, to be 4 weeks pregnant, 4 full weeks must have passed from the first day of the last normal menstruation.

There are 3 trimesters:

First   • weeks 1 to 12
Second • weeks 13 to 27
Third   • weeks 28 to 40

This book deals with the entire pregnancy and its effect on mother and baby, as well as the first 6 weeks of the baby's life, on a weekly basis. The diary also includes handy hints on lifestyle, alternative health care, practical arrangements and medical facts regarding pregnancy.

Pregnancy is a natural phase of life and the ideal opportunity for a woman to prepare herself physically and mentally for the challenge of motherhood.

A healthy lifestyle ensures that the unborn baby is protected and nurtured in order to realize its full potential.

This diary should become a treasure for the new family member, capturing precious memories of an unforgettable event.

Dr. Tilla Nicolson

first

Trimester

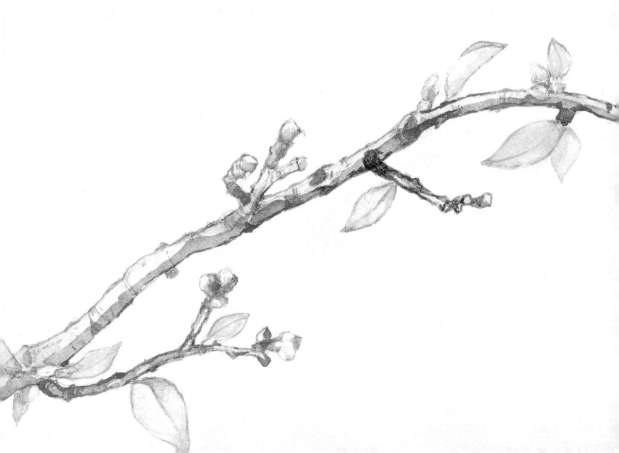

The first three months of pregnancy are undoubtedly the most important: 2 cells (a male sperm cell and a female egg cell) unite to form 1 impregnated egg cell (zygote), which then divides to become a fully developed embryo, complete with formed organs, by the end of the 12th week.

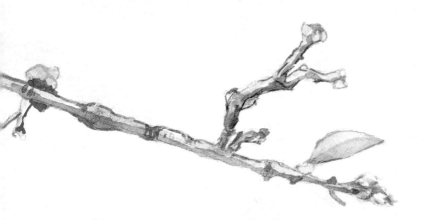

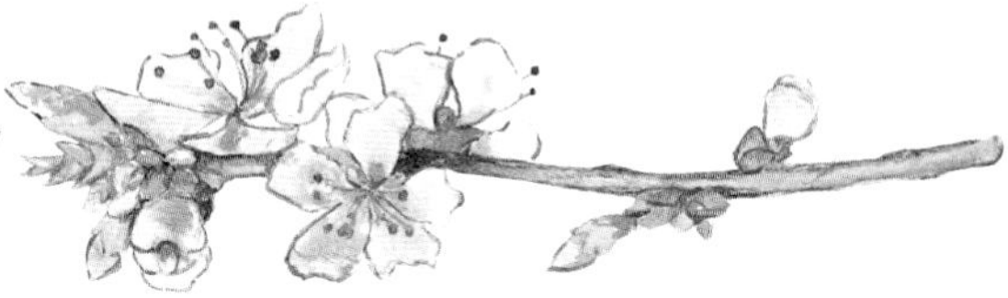

monday

tuesday

wednesday

thursday

friday

saturday

sunday

n o t e s

weight   : _____
diet   : _____
exercise   : _____
habits   : _____
next doctor's appointment: _____/_____/_____ at _____

week 1

- Optimal physical and mental health are important.
- The ideal pregnancy is a planned one.

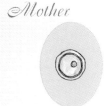

Mother

Baby

- Ovulation and conception have not yet taken place.

Lifestyle
Follow a balanced diet and do regular physical exercise. Avoid stringent diets, stop smoking and avoid or limit alcohol intake (there is no safe minimum).

Alternative hint
Pregnancy is a natural part of a woman's life. There is a worldwide tendency toward natural childbirth, breastfeeding and the holistic approach traditionally associated with midwives.

Practical hint
To accurately determine the duration of pregnancy, diarize the starting date of menstruation (see Practical hint, Week 5).

Medical hint
Ensure that you are immune to German measles (a blood test). 400 micrograms (mg) folic acid taken daily from 12 weeks before the pregnancy until the end of the first trimester reduces the incidence of neural tube defects (for example, *spina bifida* [open spine]) and cleft palate.

Discuss with your doctor the safety of taking medication for diabetes, epilepsy, asthma and heart conditions, among others. Avoid any nonessential medication, including natural medicines, unless approved by your doctor.

Avoid contact with contagious diseases.

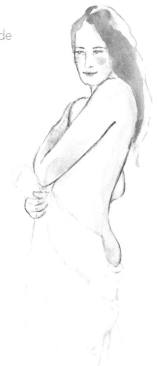

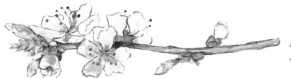

monday

tuesday

wednesday

thursday

friday

saturday

sunday

n   o   t   e   s

weight   : _____
diet   : _____
exercise   : _____
habits   : _____
next doctor's appointment: _____/_____/_____ at _____

- Ovulation takes place 12 to 16 days before the following men-struation ~ signs are, among others, a clear, thin vaginal discharge; slight rise in body temperature; a cramp (stitch) in the side and increased libido.

Mother

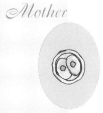

Baby

- Ovulation usually takes place in the fallopian tube around day 13 to 14 after the start of menstruation. (This is the most fertile period but conception can take place up to 5 days before and after ovulation.)
- A single sperm cell enters an ovum (egg cell) and life begins!

Lifestyle

Good health and nutrition as well as a peaceful frame of mind have a favorable effect on the development of the baby.

Alternative hint

Avoid the following aromatherapy oils during pregnancy: marjoram, pennyroyal, St. John's Wort, tansy and wormwood.

Practical hint

Formula for a boy: Repeated sex as close as possible to ovulation, following a few days of abstinence; increase sperm count by wearing loose-fitting clothes.

Formula for a girl: Sex no later than 2 days before ovulation; reduce sperm count by wearing tight-fitting underwear and having regular sex beforehand.

Medical hint

The sex of the baby is determined at the moment of conception ~ just like any other genetic factor. Theoretically the chances of having a boy or girl are 50:50, but in nature boys are slightly favored with the ratio of boys to girls being 51:49 (or 106 boys for every 100 girls).

A loving relationship

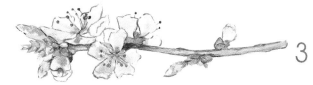

monday

tuesday

wednesday

thursday

friday

saturday

sunday

n o t e s

weight   : _____
diet   : _____
exercise   : _____
habits   : _____
next doctor's appointment: _____/_____/_____ at _____

Mother

- The uterus is not yet enlarged.
- Mostly not aware of pregnancy at all ~ could feel tired or nauseous.
- Slight vaginal bleeding (so-called *implantation bleeding*) is possible.
- Urine frequency sometimes presents as early as 1 week after conception.

Baby

- An impregnated egg cell (*zygote*) moves through the fallopian tube, rapidly divides and implants itself into the wall of the uterus 5 to 6 days after conception.
- The cells start grouping together: Some form the embryo, others the umbilical cord, placenta and amniotic sac. The nervous system and blood circulation develop first.

Lifestyle

Involve the father right from the start in planning for the new baby.

Alternative hint

An expert should be consulted for any homeopathic treatment during pregnancy. Most homeopathic remedies are safe during pregnancy, but be particularly careful up to week 12.

Practical hint

How is a new baby going to affect the mother's lifestyle, especially if she's a working mother? Financial implications are the responsibility of both parents. *Single mother:* a strong and reliable support system is of great importance.

Medical hint

It could take months to conceive ~ be patient. The fertile period is about 5 days on either side of the ovulation day.

Baby Daydream

monday

tuesday

wednesday

thursday

friday

saturday

sunday

n o t e s

weight   : _____
diet   : _____
exercise   : _____
habits   : _____
next doctor's appointment: _____/_____/_____ at _____

- Menstruation skipped ~ can therefore suspect pregnancy.
- Could have slight implantation bleeding and feel tired; breasts feel full and sensitive; may feel nauseous and have a metallic taste in the mouth.

Mother

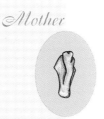

Baby

- Embryo growing rapidly.
- On day 28 he/she is visible to the naked eye.
- A tadpole-like creature with head, torso, tail and rudimentary gills.
- Precursors of all organs are formed within the first 30 days.
- Placenta starts forming.

Lifestyle

Pregnancy is not a disease. Continue with normal activities, but avoid exposure to harmful matter such as X-rays and medication.

Alternative hint

For nausea: eat regular small meals; choose fresh, unprocessed food. Camomile, peppermint and orange-blossom teas improve digestion. Ginger (fresh ginger or ginger cookies) helps with nausea.

Practical hint

A urine pregnancy test will be positive by the time menstruation is skipped (that is, 10 days after conception); a blood test is positive approximately 1 week earlier.

Medical hint

There is a 15 to 20% chance of miscarriage at this early stage. Do not get too excited or tell everybody just yet.

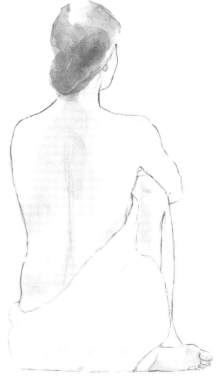

Enjoy your body

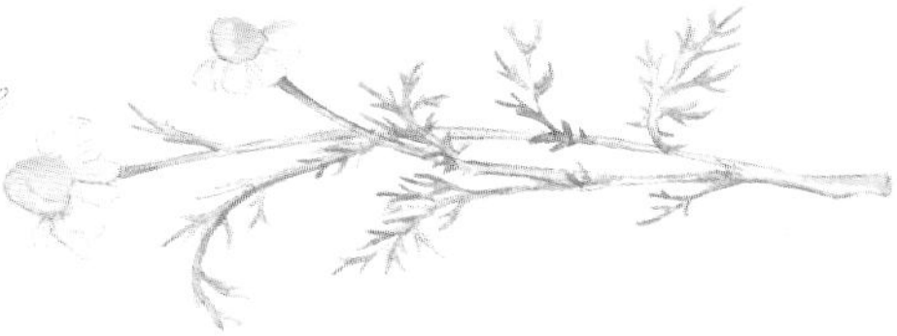

monday

tuesday

wednesday

thursday

friday

saturday

sunday

n o t e s

weight   : _____
diet   : _____
exercise   : _____
habits   : _____
next doctor's appointment: _____/_____/_____ at _____

week 5

- Menstruation skipped.
- Breasts feel tender; fatigue, nausea; bladder emptied more often.
- A metallic taste in the mouth.

Mother

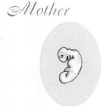

Baby

- Head and trunk are large in relation to the stumps that are to become the limbs.
- Embryo drifts in fluid-filled sac.
- Spine and brain, and a blood vessel that is to become the heart, start developing.
- Length: 0.14 inch (0.6cm); weight: .001 ounce (0.03g).

Lifestyle

Rest if you're feeling tired ~ it's normal.

Alternative hint

Massage tender breasts with 3 drops each of orange and rose oil in about half an ounce (15ml) of sweet almond oil.

Practical hint

Schedule the first prenatal visit within the next month. To determine the anticipated birth date, add 7 days to and deduct 3 months from the first day of the last normal menstruation. The date you obtain is the expected birth date in the following year.

Medical hint

Very slight implantation bleeding is normal, but consult your doctor if experiencing pain or if there is excessive bleeding. An ultrasound examination will clearly show the amniotic sac. (Heartbeat is not always visible at this stage. An ultrasound before 7 weeks could therefore cause unnecessary stress due to the absence of a heartbeat.)

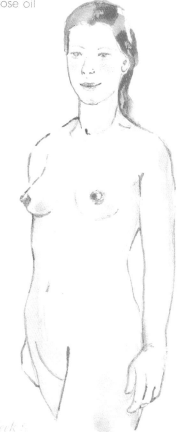

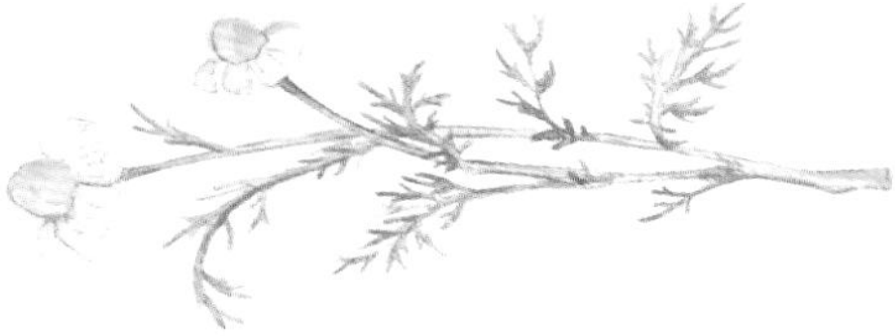

monday

tuesday

wednesday

thursday

friday

saturday

sunday

n o t e s

weight : _____
diet : _____
exercise : _____
habits : _____
next doctor's appointment: _____/_____/_____ at _____

week 6

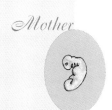

Mother

- Nausea is exacerbated by the smell of certain foods and cigarette smoke.
- Breasts become enlarged ~ stabbing pains in the breasts are normal.

Baby

- Upper and lower jaws start forming.
- The arms and then the legs start developing.
- Outer ear starts forming.
- Tubular-shaped heart starts beating and blood starts circulating.
- Digestive tract is formed.
- Sex of the embryo can be determined microscopically.

Lifestyle

Follow a good beauty routine and do not neglect personal care.

Alternative hint

Safe essential oils for aromatherapy during pregnancy are: chamomile, lavender, lemon, neroli (orange blossom), orange, rose and sandalwood.

Practical hint

Decide on the type of prenatal care and delivery:
Hospital: Doctors and nurses always available; so is medical technology.
Birth Clinic: Visit a clinic and deliver with a midwife or doctor in a home-like setting.
A home delivery by a midwife or visiting doctor can be safe if reliable resuscitation apparatus is on site.

Medical hint

Avoid medication ~ that includes herbal and over-the-counter (OTC) preparations. Worldwide, 80% of babies are delivered by midwives.

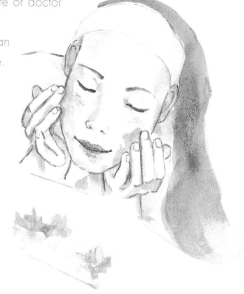

Beauty routine

monday

_____
_____
_____

tuesday

_____
_____
_____

wednesday

_____
_____
_____

thursday

_____
_____
_____

friday

_____
_____
_____

saturday

_____
_____
_____

sunday

_____
_____
_____

n   o   t   e   s

weight   : _____
diet   : _____
exercise   : _____
habits   : _____
next doctor's appointment: _____/_____/_____ at _____

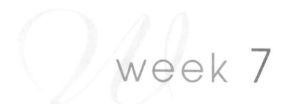

week 7

- Overwhelming fatigue.
- Sex drive could diminish (but will return in the second trimester).

Mother

Baby

- Brain develops; he/she is growing rapidly. • Movement takes place, but is too weak to be felt.
- Hands start forming.
- Arms and legs split at the ends (future fingers and toes).
- Heartbeat can be seen on ultrasound. • Bone cells start developing. • Length: .52 inch (1.3cm); weight: .028oz (0.8g).

Lifestyle

You may experience a wide range of emotions while adjusting to the thought of being pregnant.

Reinforce your relationship with your husband or partner ~ communicate, share your feelings and listen to one another.

Alternative hint

Chamomile tea has a calming effect and improves sleep and digestion.

Practical hint

Financial planning for baby: Do not buy too much too soon.
Where possible, borrow from friends or family.

Medical hint

If bleeding occurs, consult a doctor to eliminate the possibility of a tubal pregnancy or miscarriage.
Early miscarriages due to abnormal development are not due to human error and therefore not the mother's fault!

Rest if you feel tired

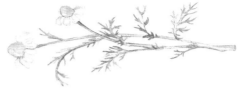

monday

tuesday

wednesday

thursday

friday

saturday

sunday

n   o   t   e   s

weight   : _____

diet   :

exercise   :

habits   :

next doctor's appointment: _____/_____/_____ at _____

week 8

- Still feels nauseous and tired.
- Breasts continue enlarging.
- Very emotional.
- Increased vaginal discharge.

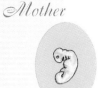

Mother

Baby

- Wrists and elbows discernible.
- Fingers, inner ears and eyes start forming.
- Umbilical cord has formed.
- Has a little tail.
- Length: 1.2 inches (3.2cm); weight: .035oz (1g).

Lifestyle
A balanced diet and regular exercise ease constipation and mood swings. Guard against excessive weight gain ~ maximum 5.5 pounds (2.5kg) in the first trimester (may even lose weight from nausea).

Alternative hint
Nettle tea is rich in iron, purifies the blood and is an excellent tonic during pregnancy.

Practical hint
A single parent in particular should do proper planning for after the baby's birth. Will there be financial assistance from the other parent? Join a support group if necessary.

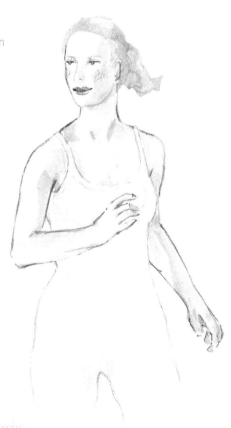

Medical hint
Embryo now very susceptible to developmental and hormonal defects.
Medical fact: 1 in 5 early pregnancies could end in miscarriage.

Regular exercise

monday

....
....
....

tuesday

....
....
....

wednesday

....
....
....

thursday

....
....
....

friday

....
....
....

saturday

....
....
....

sunday

....
....
....

n o t e s

weight   : _____
diet   : _____
exercise   : _____
habits   : _____
next doctor's appointment: _____/_____/_____ at _____

Mother

- Starts gaining weight.
- Gums are softer and swollen.
- Starts getting adjusted to the idea of pregnancy and motherhood, even though it seems unreal.

Baby

- Now called a *fetus*. • Reacts to stimulation: feet kick, toes curl, makes a fist, frowns, opens mouth.
- Webbed fingers visible and longer.
- Toes visible, little tail disappears.
- Skin thickens: hair follicles, muscles, bone tissue and teeth start deve-loping. Ears develop.
- Eyes open and developed.

Lifestyle

Oral hygiene and regular dental checkups are very important. Gather information on pregnancy. In a first pregnancy this will prevent unnecessary fears and surprises.

Alternative hint

Relax in an aromatherapy bath: Add 3 to 4 drops of essential oil such as sandalwood, lavender, lemon grass, rose, jasmine, lemon or bergamot to bath water.
Important: Avoid marjoram, sage, thyme and wintergreen during pregnancy.

Practical hint

Make a dental appointment.
Seek genetic counseling if there are any chromosome abnormalities in the family, if there is a history of spina bifida, deafness or blindness, if you have had more than 3 inexplicable miscarriages, or if you are over 35 years old.

Medical hint

Women who are underweight by 15% or more at the time of conception have an increased incidence of babies with low birth weight, pre-eclampsia (high blood pressure) and premature birth.

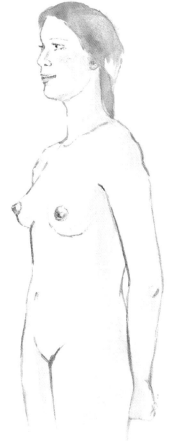

monday

....
....
....

tuesday

....
....
....

wednesday

....
....
....

thursday

....
....
....

friday

....
....
....

saturday

....
....
....

sunday

....
....
....

n o t e s

weight   : _____
diet   : _____
exercise   : _____
habits   : _____
next doctor's appointment: _____/_____/_____ at _____

- Emotional.
- Blood volume increases by 40 to 45% ~ sufficient iron intake is therefore necessary to prevent anemia (low red blood cell count).

Mother

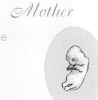

Baby

- Eyelids sealed by the end of the week.
- Head still large, but looks like a human being.
- Limbs are short and thin.
- At the end of week 10: All organs present and fully formed, including the kidneys.
- Length: 1.8 inches (4.5cm); weight: .18oz (5g).

Lifestyle

Couvade syndrome: The expecting father develops nausea, gains weight, has food cravings and becomes emotionally unstable ~ in sympathy with his wife!
Depending on their age, involve other children as much as possible in the pregnancy.

Alternative hint

Drink herbal teas that do not affect iron absorption and contain no caffeine, instead of tea or coffee.

Practical hint

Obtain information on maternity benefits at work.
Inform employer of your pregnancy.
Travel is allowed, but avoid malaria areas.
The second trimester is the best time for traveling.
Always wear a seatbelt in the car.

Medical hint

Excessive alcohol intake leads to fetal alcohol syndrome, accompanied by stunted growth and mental retardation. There is no safe minimum alcohol intake. Cigarette smoke could retard growth and adversely affects reading and arithmetic capabilities. Avoid passive smoking.

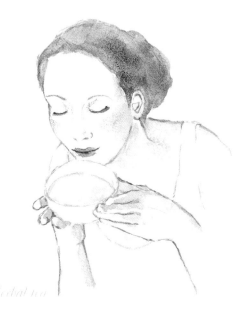

Herbal tea

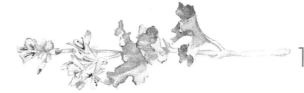

monday

tuesday

wednesday

thursday

friday

saturday

sunday

n o t e s

weight   : _____
diet   : _____
exercise   : _____
habits   : _____
next doctor's appointment: _____/_____/_____ at _____

week 11

- Starts feeling less tired and nauseous.
- Breast changes become obvious.

Mother

Baby

- Small quantities of urine are discharged.
- Until now the external sex organs of both sexes have looked the same.
- Length: 2.2 inches (5.5cm); weight: .35oz (10g).

Lifestyle

Replace fatty foods with health foods. Eat several small meals a day; eat slowly. Diet must be balanced ~ you need an extra 125 calories a day = 500ml low-fat milk or a whole-wheat sandwich with a protein filling. *Vegetarian diet:* vitamin B12 supplement is required if you do not eat any animal products.

Alternative hint

For nausea: herbal tea (ginger or camomile) and a dry cracker 30 minutes before getting up; another cup of herbal tea 30 minutes later with a slice of whole-wheat toast.

Practical hint

Follow-up visits during pregnancy: Monthly up to 32 weeks; twice a month up to 36 weeks and then weekly, but varies according to risk level of pregnancy.

Medical hint

Conditions that could hamper normal development (for example, viral diseases and toxins) reveal their harmful effects before week 12. 70% of women feel nauseous or queasy between 4 and 14 weeks. This is linked to good fetal health. Avoid handling cats (particularly sick cats and sandboxes), because infection by toxoplasmosis (treatable), prevalent in cats, causes mental retardation, epilepsy and blindness in babies.

Eat healthful

monday

tuesday

wednesday

thursday

friday

saturday

sunday

n o t e s

weight   : _____
diet   : _____
exercise   : _____
habits   : _____
next doctor's appointment: _____/_____/_____ at _____

- Nausea much less.
- Uterus can be felt above edge of pelvis.
- Pigmentation marks could appear on face.
- Breasts: Clear surface blood vessels; nipples larger and darker.

Mother

Baby

- Lies curled up with chin drawn in and knees pulled up.
- Sentient, feeling being.
- Little heart races if mother becomes excited or anxious.
- Length: 3 inches (7.5cm); weight: .98oz (28g).

Lifestyle

Maternal stress, particularly grief, retards fetal development.

Persistent stress causes fetus to be restless and impairs development.

Hair (on the scalp) increases during pregnancy ~ falls out afterward.

Alternative hint

Relax ~ it calms the fetus and promotes growth and development. Acquired techniques under an expert's guidance, such as yoga and meditation, are useful and safe.

Practical hint

Floss and brush teeth regularly. Sunscreen limits pigmentation.

Medical hint

Chances of a miscarriage are decreasing.

Two-thirds of serious abnormalities can be detected prenatally. Screening tests such as ultrasound and blood tests are used to determine the risk of abnormalities. Diagnostic tests such as amniocentesis for Down syndrome are more invasive, but provide conclusive answers. Sonar examination at 11 to 13 weeks can determine fetal age and presence of certain abnormalities, while measurement of fat cushion behind neck can determine presence of Down syndrome (often combined with a blood test at about 16 weeks).

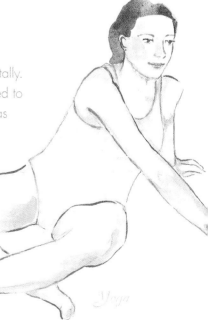

Yoga

second

Trimester

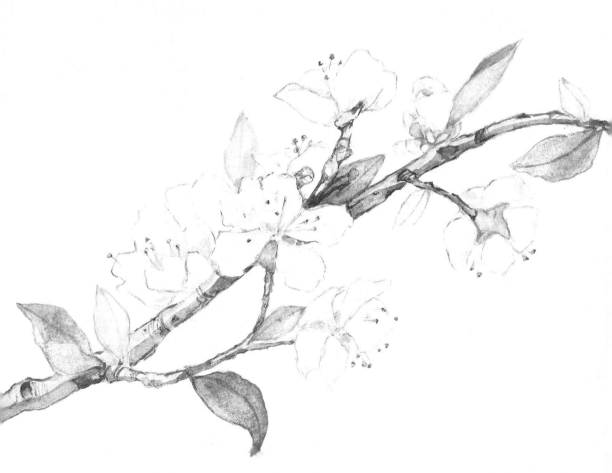

Nausea and fatigue improve. The important developmental phase is over. The second trimester is the honeymoon phase of pregnancy. Enjoy every moment!

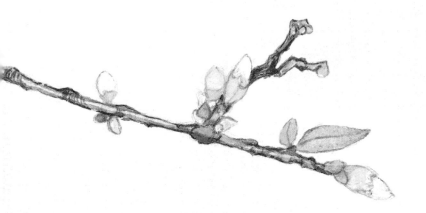

monday

tuesday

wednesday

thursday

friday

saturday

sunday

n   o   t   e   s

weight   : _____
diet   : _____
exercise   : _____
habits   : _____
next doctor's appointment: _____/_____/_____ at _____

week 13

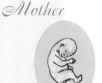

- Feels good ~ no longer so tired.
- Enjoys pregnancy.
- Nausea starts to improve.

Mother

Baby

- Moves freely in approximately 3.4 oz (100 ml) amniotic fluid.
- Grows rapidly.
- Bone marrow, liver and spleen produce blood cells.
- Bone structure developed and teeth formed.
- Length: 3 inches (7.5cm); weight: 1.05oz (30g).

Lifestyle

Exercise 15 to 30 minutes a day, 3 to 4 times a week.
Maximum pulse rate: 120 to 140 beats a minute (must be able to have a conversation).
Pain is a warning signal. Avoid dangerous exercise such as skiing,
skateboarding or horse-riding. Swimming is the ideal exercise.

Alternative hint

For constipation: Exercise, high liquid intake and prunes,
soaked in water overnight (drink the juice as well).

Practice hint

Nature prepares the breasts for breastfeeding.
Wear a good support bra. Expose nipples to the sun for 5
minutes a day. Are nipples inverted? Squeeze on either side
of the nipple with thumb and forefinger ~ if there is an
indentation, stretching exercises of the nipple (Hoffman
exercises) should be done daily. A nipple cap can also be
worn for a few hours a day.

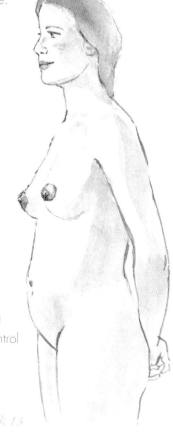

Medical hint

Weight gain of approximately two-thirds of a pound (0.4 kg)
a week up to the end of pregnancy is ideal. Blood-sugar control
is essential for diabetics ~ the second trimester is particularly
critical, and therefore strict prenatal care is essential.

monday

tuesday

wednesday

thursday

friday

saturday

sunday

n o t e s

weight   : _____
diet   : _____
exercise   : _____
habits   : _____
next doctor's appointment: _____/_____/_____ at _____

Mother

- Feels much better ~ experiences increased libido ("honeymoon phase").
- May want to experiment with different positions to make sex more comfortable.

- Sex clearly discernible.
- Heartbeat audible with ultrasound.
- Chin, forehead and nose clearly visible ~ can turn head.
- Length: 3.6 inches (9cm); weight: 2.1oz (60g).

Baby

Lifestyle

More comfortable sleeping on the side.

Sex is safe, unless advised by a medical doctor to be cautious.

Experiment with different positions ~ do not place weight on the baby.

Baby is well-protected in amniotic sac.

Alternative hint

For varicose veins: Do not squat or stand for long periods at a time or cross your legs when you sit. Do regular exercises. Raw garlic, onions and parsley increase the elasticity of the blood vessels. Try witch hazel drops or ointment.

Practical hint

Arrange maternity leave and discuss who will be responsible for work done in your absence. Buy good support bras.

Medical hint

If still plagued by varicose veins: Wear special stockings and keep the legs raised as much as possible when sitting and sleeping. Discomfort will probably increase as the pregnancy progresses.

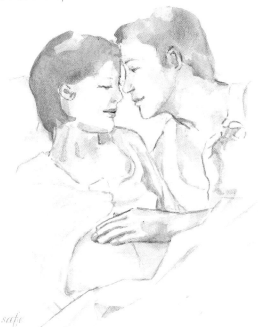

Sex is safe

monday

tuesday

wednesday

thursday

friday

saturday

sunday

n o t e s

weight : _____
diet : _____
exercise : _____
habits : _____
next doctor's appointment: _____/_____/_____ at _____

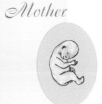

- Feels well and energetic.
- Could be plagued by lower backache and hemorrhoids could be a bother.
- Increased vaginal discharge can be a problem.

Mother

Baby

- Makes breathing movements.
- Skeleton developed ~ legs longer than arms.
- Can hear.
- Length: 4.8 inches (12cm); weight: 3.5oz (100g).

Lifestyle

Protect the back by bending the knees when lifting objects. Strengthen stomach muscles (exercise) to protect the back.

Alternative hint

Prenatal stimulation of the baby with soft classical music could make the baby calmer after birth. (This is not essential, however.)

Practical hint

A pregnant woman is prone to bladder infections and vaginal thrush (candidiasis). Wear only cotton underwear and use only white toilet paper. Showering is preferable to bathing.

Medical hint

Moderate swelling of the ankles is normal, provided the blood pressure is normal.

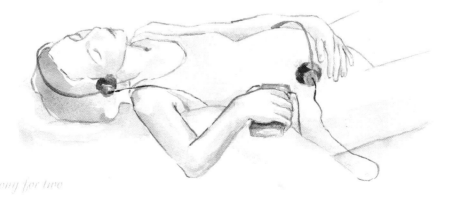

Symphony for two

monday

tuesday

wednesday

thursday

friday

saturday

sunday

n o t e s

weight : _____
diet : _____
exercise : _____
habits : _____
next doctor's appointment: _____/_____/_____ at _____

- In second and subsequent pregnancies, mother may now possibly feel the baby move inside.
- Stomach can no longer be hidden; uterus halfway between upper edge of pelvis and navel.
- Linea nigra (pigmented line) appears on stomach.
- Stretch marks may start appearing.

Mother

Baby

- Hair, eyelashes and eyebrows start growing.
- Soft finger and toenails start forming.
- Fetus has a neck.
- Small nipples appear.
- Entire body covered with fine down.
- Length: 6 inches (15cm); weight: 4oz (114g).

Lifestyle

Avoid tight-fitting clothes.

Guard against excessive weight gain.

Think carefully before having an amniocentesis (if indicated) ~ the results may require you to make a decision. A needle is inserted into the uterus through the pelvic wall and a sample of amniotic fluid is drawn for analysis. It is a sterile procedure and the results are obtained within about 4 weeks. Amniocentesis holds a 1% risk of miscarriage.

Alternative hint

For heartburn: Avoid large evening meals; chew mint leaves; a fennel infusion improves digestion.

Practical hint

Amniocentesis is done at 16 to 18 weeks to establish if there are any chromosomal abnormalities in women over the age of 35, or after an abnormal triple blood test (the latter is done at 15 to 18 weeks).

Medical hint

Some diseases, such as German measles, can harm the fetus, particularly those involving a high fever, such as malaria, which could induce labor, so inform your doctor right away if you feel unwell.

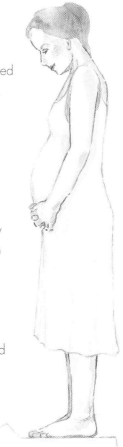

Keep an eye on your weight

Lemon blossom

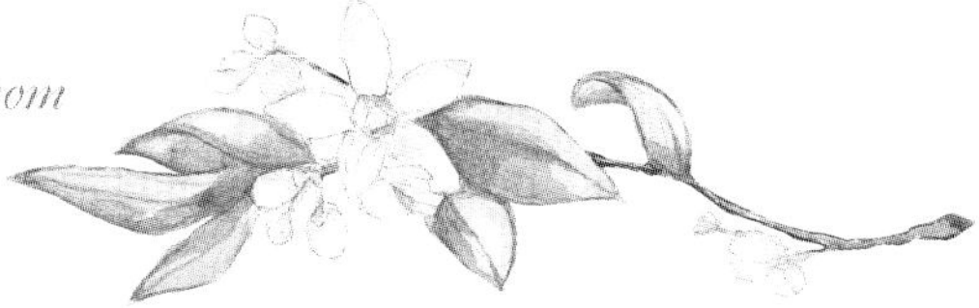

monday

tuesday

wednesday

thursday

friday

saturday

sunday

n o t e s

weight : ________

diet : ____

exercise : ____

habits : ____

next doctor's appointment: ____/____/____ at ________

- Waistline has disappeared.
- Feels good.
- Feels positive about the pregnancy and getting used to the idea of having a baby.

Mother

Baby

- Limbs, skin and bone structure fully developed.
- Can discern sweet and other tastes.
- Length: 7.2 inches (18cm); weight: 6.5oz (185g).

Lifestyle

Dress stylishly to boost spirits and feel more feminine!
For the first 7 months, ordinary loose-fitting clothes are acceptable.
Wear simple, comfortable clothes and fashionable, flat shoes.

Alternative hint

A stuffy nose is common during pregnancy.
Try saline nose drops or homeopathic drops.

Practical hint

Start buying a package of disposable diapers (for newborns)
each month ~ to make life easier the first few days after
the birth.

Medical hint

20 to 50% of pregnant women develop hemorrhoids
with slight bleeding.
Prevent constipation by exercising, drinking plenty
of liquids, and eating plenty of fresh fruit and
vegetables.
Use a special ointment to lessen the pain, if necessary.

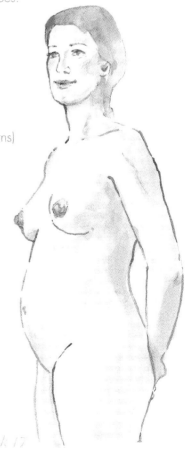

18

monday

tuesday

wednesday

thursday

friday

saturday

sunday

n o t e s

weight : _____
diet : _____
exercise : _____
habits : _____
next doctor's appointment: _____/_____/_____ at _____

week 18

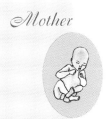

Mother

- In first pregnancy, first movements are felt now ~ exciting!
- Stuffy nose (common).
- Increased vaginal discharge.
- Hair texture could change.
- Pigmentation marks on face, aggravated by sunlight.

Baby

- Approximately 0.35 oz (10 to 20ml) urine discharged and the same amount of amniotic fluid swallowed a day.
- Can hear ~ alarmed by sudden noises.
- Length: 8.4 inches (21cm); weight: 8.2oz (235g).

Lifestyle

Try to look your best ~ pay extra attention to clothes, make-up and general care. Looking good makes you feel better.

Alternative hint

Nettle tea relieves muscle cramps in legs, as do other homeopathic remedies.

Practical hint

Start buying baby's layette, but be judicious ~ beware of temptations in baby stores. Involve the father and other children.

Medical hint

Average time between feeling the first movement and birth is 147 days. Diarize the date.

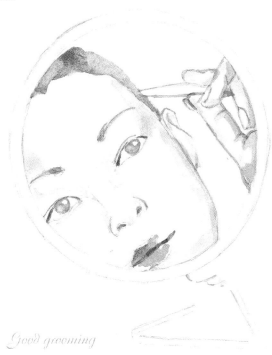

Good grooming

monday

tuesday

wednesday

thursday

friday

saturday

sunday

notes

weight : _____
diet : _____
exercise : _____
habits : _____
next doctor's appointment: _____/_____/_____ at _____

- Extra weight on hips, thighs and stomach.
- Braxton-Hicks contractions ("practice contractions") often follow movement by the baby.

Mother

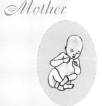

Baby

- Baby teeth are developed in gums, and buds for permanent teeth start forming.
- Length: 9.2 inches (23cm); weight: 10oz (285g).

Lifestyle

Foot care is important because the feet are carrying more and more weight.
Wear comfortable shoes.
Regular pedicures and foot spas work wonders!

Alternative hint

Massage feet and swollen ankles with 2 drops each of benzoin, rose and neroli oils in half an ounce (15ml) sesame-seed oil.

Practical hint

Do you want to know the sex of your baby beforehand? Inform the person doing the ultrasound examination of your decision (around weeks 18 to 22).

Medical hint

Don't worry about possible abnormalities because 99% of all babies are normal at birth.
The baby is attached to the placenta by an umbilical cord. The placenta provides nutrition, breathing, secretion, hormones and enzymes.

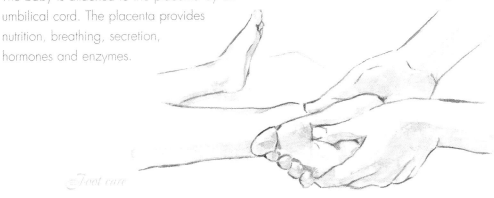

Foot care

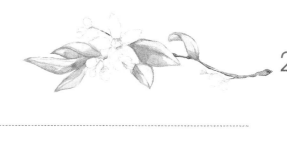

2 0

monday

tuesday

wednesday

thursday

friday

saturday

sunday

n o t e s

weight   : _____
diet   : _____
exercise   : _____
habits   : _____
next doctor's appointment: _____/_____/_____ at _____

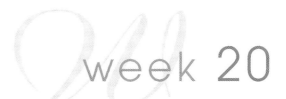

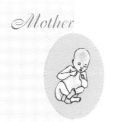

Mother

- Uterus now at the navel.
- Heartburn common.
- Nails grow more rapidly and stronger, but sometimes more brittle.

Baby

- Skin less translucent; covered in fine down (lanugo) and water-permeable. • Eyelids still closed, ears visible. • Hair starts growing on head. • Lungs solid. • Starts looking like a baby; thin, due to lack of subcutaneous fat.
- Length: 10 inches (25cm); weight: 10.5oz (300g).

Lifestyle

As uterus enlarges, your center of gravity shifts. Take this into account when moving around ~ it is easier to fall, so take care! Let your children and partner feel the baby kicking. They could also attend the ultrasound test.

Alternative hint

Keep abdominal skin supple by massaging with 5 drops of aromatic lavender oil in half an ounce (15ml) jojoba, wheat germ or evening primrose oil. Continue daily until after the birth. Guard against sudden, excessive weight gain.

Practical hint

For hospital delivery: Find out whether you have to make a reservation; arrange a visit to the maternity ward.

Medical hint

An ultrasound evaluates fetal growth and detects neural-tube defects, cleft palate and heart and kidney abnormalities. Baby's sex can also easily be seen.

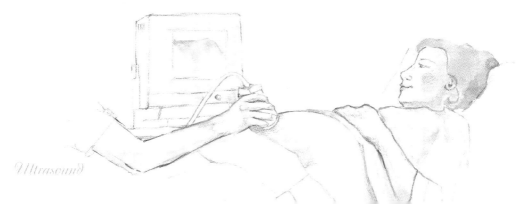

Ultrasound

Peppermint

2 1

monday

tuesday

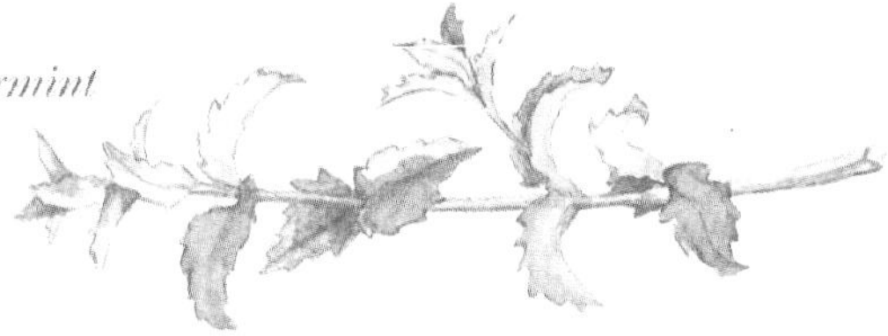

wednesday

thursday

friday

saturday

sunday

n o t e s

weight : ________

diet : ____

exercise : ____

habits : ____

next doctor's appointment: _____/_____/_____ at _________

- Sees abdominal wall move when baby kicks.
- Feels energetic.
- Heartburn, swollen ankles, sleep disturbances.
- Breasts start producing milk (colostrum).

Mother

- Very active.
- Becomes calm if mother speaks softly or rubs over the uterus.
- Length: 11.2 inches (28cm); weight: 13.7oz (390g).

Baby

Lifestyle

Good posture reduces backache and a healthful diet increases energy levels.

Alternative hint

Massage relieves pain and muscle spasms. Ask your partner to give you a massage or arrange for a full body massage at a beauty salon.
Self-massage: Place your hands on your shoulders and press down firmly. Rest palms and fingers on the shoulders and circulate fingers behind shoulders.

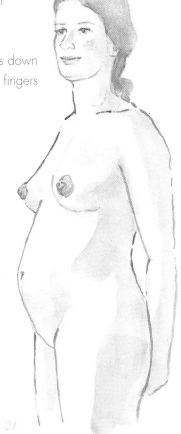

Practical hint

Baby's crib must be safe; use lead-free, nontoxic paint or varnish.
Stroller: Large wheels are more suitable for uneven terrain; it must be collapsible if you often travel by car.

Medical hint

Breast size does not influence the ability to breastfeed. Only 1% of women produce insufficient breast milk.

monday

_____
_____
_____

tuesday

_____
_____
_____

wednesday

_____
_____
_____

thursday

_____
_____
_____

friday

_____
_____
_____

saturday

_____
_____
_____

sunday

_____
_____
_____

n o t e s

weight   : _____
diet   : _____
exercise   : _____
habits   : _____
next doctor's appointment: _____/_____/_____ at _____

- Feels good and enjoys pregnancy.
- Weight gain now about 14 ounces (400g) a week.

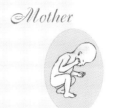

Mother

Baby

- Nostrils and alveoli (air sacs) in the lungs start developing.
- Length: 11.8 inches (29.5cm); weight: 14.7oz (420g).

Lifestyle

More than 60% of mothers work; make all the arrangements now for care of the baby after maternity leave.

Alternative hint

Walking, yoga, swimming and water aerobics are ideal. Prenatal classes are strongly recommended ~ they provide you with knowledge of all the options during your pregnancy and help you and your partner to make informed decisions that are best for you.

Practical hint

Invest in a baby seat for the car that complies with federal safety standards.
Note: An airbag on the passenger side of a car could be potentially dangerous to baby. Put baby seat in center of back seat.

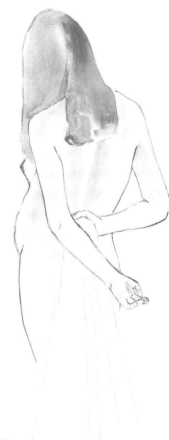

Medical hint

Rhesus-incompatibility: If mother is Rh-negative and father Rh-positive, baby could be Rh-positive and mother could develop antibodies against baby. A prenatal blood test is done to check for antibodies; after the birth a Rhogam® (anti-D-immunoglobulin) is injected into the mother to destroy anti-bodies; may also be administered during pregnancy.

Spoil yourself

monday

tuesday

wednesday

thursday

friday

saturday

sunday

n   o   t   e   s

weight   : _____
diet   : _____
exercise   : _____
habits   : _____
next doctor's appointment: _____/_____/_____ at _____

- May feel a stabbing pain in side ~ caused by the round ligament stretching (not harmful, disappears with rest).
- It is normal to pass urine frequently.

Mother

Baby

- Starts looking like a baby.
- *Boy:* scrotum well developed.
- *Girl:* ovaries contain millions of eggs (reducing to 2 million at birth).
- Length: 12.4 inches (31cm); weight: 15.4oz (440g).

Lifestyle

A pregnant woman is susceptible to bladder infections; to prevent this, empty the bladder regularly and drink at least 8 glasses of water a day.

Alternative hint

Acupuncture could relieve backache, but must be administered by an expert ~ and with great care!

Practical hint

Prepare baby's room as follows:

- Simple, safe, warm. • Dim night light.
- Bed for baby and work surface preferably at a comfortable height.
- Baby must not sleep directly under a window or near an air conditioner.
- A chair for breastfeeding is convenient.

Medical hint

Check blood pressure regularly: Pre-eclampsia is high blood pressure with protein in the urine after 20 weeks of pregnancy. This could lead to eclampsia in the mother and may be dangerous to the baby.
Warning signals: severe headache, blurred vision, sudden weight gain, and swollen ankles, hands and face.

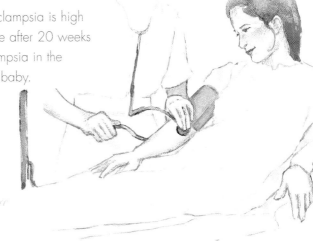

Check blood pressure

monday

tuesday

wednesday

thursday

friday

saturday

sunday

n o t e s

weight : _____
diet : _____
exercise : _____
habits : _____
next doctor's appointment: _____/_____/_____ at _____

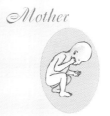

Mother

- Should be feeling strong signs of life.
- Workload of heart now 35% higher.
- Pulse rate 15 to 20 beats a minute faster than before pregnancy.

Baby

- Limbs have muscles, but weak and thin.
- Reacts to loud noises, senses rhythm of music.
- Skin thickens and becomes non-translucent.
- Develops sleep-and-waking pattern.
- Length: 13.2 inches (33cm); weight: 17.5oz (500g).

Lifestyle

Relaxation technique: Lie comfortably on back or side, propped by pillows. Close your eyes and focus on your breathing ~ regulated exhaling is particularly important: Exhale slowly. Now start at the feet: contract muscles and relax. Move upward through the body: Contract and relax. Remember shoulders and jaw. Empty your mind and focus on a peaceful image.

Practical hint

Baby's requirements: safe place to sleep; 3 to 4 sheets (plus a waterproof sheet); 1 to 2 thick and 2 thinner blankets; 2 towels and a washcloth; baby soap, shampoo, cream and ointment; diapers: disposable (initially about 10 a day) or towelling (at least 10 to 15), diaper linings, diaper pins, diaper pail and sterilizing liquid, 4 plastic waterproofs; for bottle-feeding: 2 to 6 bottles with nipples, bottle brush and baby milk; 6 "onesies" (or 4 with 2 sets of pajamas); 2 rompers and pairs of socks; 4 bibs; hat (if cold), hair brush, nail scissors. Always dress baby in one more layer of clothes than mother - newborn babies lose heat easily, and should be dressed warmly.

Medical hint

1 in 80 pregnancies are twins. Discomfort during pregnancy is worse, which makes rest, a balanced diet and good prenatal medical care extremely important.

Aromatherapy bath

monday

....
....
....

tuesday

....
....
....

wednesday

....
....
....

thursday

....
....
....

friday

....
....
....

saturday

....
....
....

sunday

....
....
....

n   o   t   e   s

weight   : _____
diet   : _____
exercise   : _____
habits   : _____
next doctor's appointment: _____/_____/_____ at _____

- Feels healthy; increased pressure on bladder (goes to the toilet regularly).
- Muscle spasms are common, particularly at night.

Mother

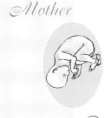

Baby

- Body covered with waxy substance called *vernix*.
- Down on body becomes less, but more hair on head (many babies are bald).
- Sucks thumb; has hiccups (practices breathing and swallows amniotic fluid).
- Length: 13.6 inches (34cm); weight: 21oz (600g).

Lifestyle

Discuss the father's fears about the impending birth ~ the biggest fear is often that you won't get to the hospital on time!

Alternative hint

Muscle spasms: Prevent them by doing regular exercise and taking a calcium and magnesium supplement.
Stretch the muscle when it goes into spasm.

Practical hint

Breastfeeding or bottle-feeding? Breast milk is the best baby food and it is free! It also protects baby against infections and allergies.
Bottle-feeding: You will need about 6 bottles (4 ounces/125ml), a bottlebrush, sterilizing liquid and 1 can of formula milk (for newborns).

Medical hint

Do not wash nipples with soap; it dries out the skin and causes them to crack. Use a little colostrum for massaging the nipples ~ they should be soft and pliable.

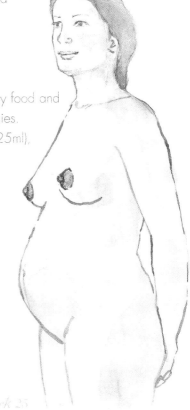

monday

----

tuesday

----

wednesday

----

thursday

----

friday

----

saturday

----

sunday

----

n   o   t   e   s

weight   : _____
diet   : _____
exercise   : _____
habits   : _____
next doctor's appointment: _____/_____/_____ at _____

Mother

- Braxton-Hicks contractions (not painful) now more common.
- Heartburn and backache common.
- May experience sleeping difficulties.

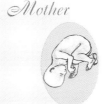

Baby

- Eyes open; has eyelashes, eyebrows.
- Has fingerprints. • Strong enough grip to support own weight. • Starts depositing subcutaneous fat, which helps regulate body temperature.
- Amniotic fluid volume: about 1 liter.
- Length: 14 inches (35cm); weight: 24.5oz (700g).

Lifestyle

Common fears:

- Will I be a good mother?
- Will the baby be normal?
- Will I love the baby as much as I love my other child(ren)?

If you are well prepared and armed with sufficient knowledge, you will feel confident, come what may.

Alternative hint

Be careful when taking general multivitamin supplements ~ more than 5,000 IU of vitamin A daily could lead to abnormalities in the baby. Pregnancy multivitamin supplements are safe in the recommended doses.

Practical hint

Decide on date for maternity leave in consultation with employer. Arrange prenatal classes (if available).

Medical hint

If you have doubts about the baby's well-being, lie on your left side and count the number of movements you feel in 1 hour. If there are fewer than 10 an hour, repeat, and if there are still fewer than 10 movements an hour, consult your doctor.

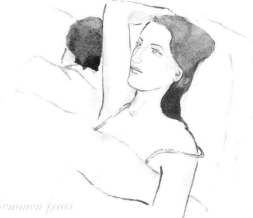

Common fears

monday

....
....
....

tuesday

....
....
....

wednesday

....
....
....

thursday

....
....
....

friday

....
....
....

saturday

....
....
....

sunday

....
....
....

n o t e s

weight   : _____
diet   : _____
exercise : _____
habits   : _____
next doctor's appointment: _____/_____/_____ at _____

- Uterus now much larger.
- Blood pressure reaches a low; may feel tired and listless.
- Baby's movements tend to be more active while mother is sleeping.

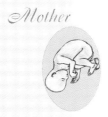

Mother

Baby

- Eyes open ~ sees light through abdominal wall.
- Starts sucking ~ even thumb or fist!
- Length: 14.4 inches (36cm); weight: 28 oz (800g).

Lifestyle

Avoid sleeping on your back because blood pressure drops due to pressure of uterus on blood vessels. Instead, sleep on your left side.

Practical hint

Choices of delivery:

Natural: no medical intervention.

Water birth: birth partly in water for pain relief (a special spa bath is often used).

Active birth: walk around during birth ~ gravity speeds up the process.

Medically assisted delivery: medical intervention, induction, pain relief, episiotomy, etc.

Cesarean section: baby is delivered through a section in the abdominal wall and uterus.

Medical hint

Ensure adequate iron intake. Check hemoglobin levels ~ daily supplement of 18 to 30mg of iron required during pregnancy and breastfeeding.

Good sources: liver, meat, eggs, whole-wheat bread and raisins.

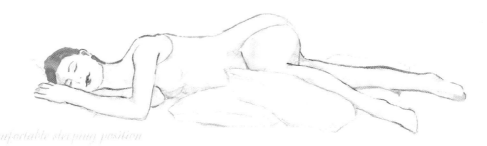

Comfortable sleeping position

third

Trimester

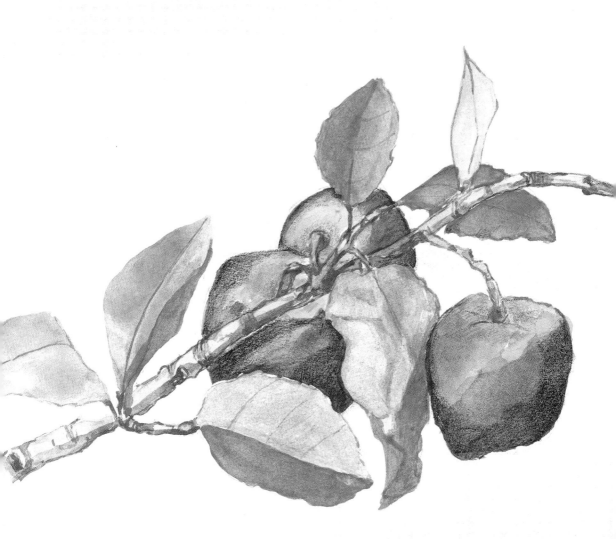

Physical discomfort increases ~ as well as anxiety and fear of the impending birth. Mother experiences a strong protective feeling toward baby.

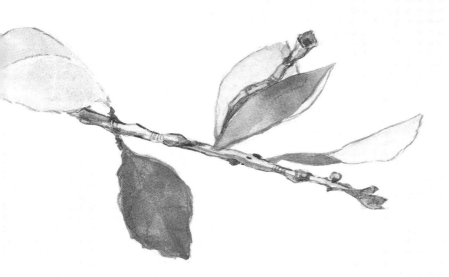

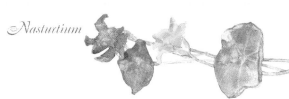

Nasturtium

monday

tuesday

wednesday

thursday

friday

saturday

sunday

n o t e s

weight : _____
diet : _____
exercise : _____
habits : _____
next doctor's appointment: _____/_____/_____ at _____

- Breasts produce colostrum.
- Although you may feel short of breath, the oxygen capacity of the lungs is 20% higher than when not pregnant.

Mother

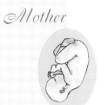

Baby

- Lungs still immature.
- Heartbeat approximately 150 beats a minute.
- Length: 14.8 inches (37cm); weight: 31.5oz (900g).

Lifestyle

Pelvic floor exercises improve bladder control before and after the birth. Tightly contract muscles that control the bladder for as long as possible ~ repeat approximately 10 times a day.

Alternative hint

Keep hips, pelvis and lower back supple by regularly sitting on the floor with legs crossed (knees and hips bent).

Practical hint

Draw up a birth plan and decide on a companion.
Take into account: • Where you want to have the birth.
• Role of the companion (also during intervention or Cesarean). • Position during delivery and birth.
• Procedures you would like to avoid. • Pain relief (if any). • Feelings about use of forceps or suction.
• Special needs. • Whether you want to hold the baby immediately. • Care of the baby immediately after the birth. Remember, everything does not always go according to plan.

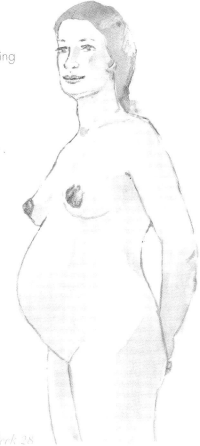

Medical hint

Premature baby has a good chance of survival if born now and placed in a special neonatal unit.

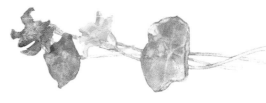

monday

tuesday

wednesday

thursday

friday

saturday

sunday

n o t e s

weight : _____
diet : _____
exercise : _____
habits : _____
next doctor's appointment: _____/_____/_____ at _____

- Uncomfortable and tired ~ you need more rest.
- Increased urination frequency; regular backache and heartburn.

Mother

- Skin red and wrinkled; subcutaneous fat starts forming.
- Eyes can blink and start focusing.
- Length: approximately 15 inches (38cm); weight 2.2lb (1kg).

Baby

Lifestyle

50% of women develop stretchmarks. Determined by type and suppleness of skin. Guard against sudden weight gain.

Alternative hint

Massaging abdominal skin with aromatherapy oils (5 drops in half an ounce [15ml] jojoba, wheat germ or evening primrose oil) is soothing, but probably not that effective in preventing stretchmarks.

Practical hint

Start thinking of possible names for baby ~ Do not underestimate the importance of this decision; the child has to live with it for the rest of his or her life!

Medical hint

Vaginal bleeding should always be regarded as potentially serious: • Low-lying placenta (*placenta previa*) causes painless bleeding (repeated) and is usually not dangerous.

• Detachment of the placenta (*placental abruption*) causes painful contraction of the uterus and bleeding, and is the most common cause of fetal death. Inform your doctor immediately.

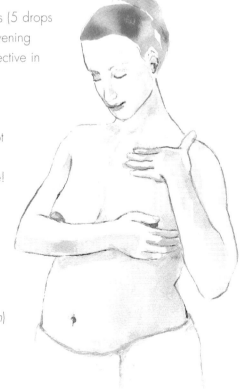

Stretchmark prevention

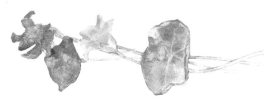

30

monday

....
....
....

tuesday

....
....
....

wednesday

....
....
....

thursday

....
....
....

friday

....
....
....

saturday

....
....
....

sunday

....
....
....

n   o   t   e   s

weight   : _____
diet   : _____
exercise   : _____
habits   : _____
next doctor's appointment: _____/_____/_____ at _____

Mother

- Backache and sleep disturbances common.
- Uterus halfway between navel and bottom of breastbone; navel now flat.

- Moves actively.
- Length: 15.6 inches (39cm); weight: 2.42lb (1.1kg).

Baby

Lifestyle

Travel is allowed ~ Discuss long trips with your doctor or midwife. Cut-off point on international airlines is commonly 32 weeks. For local air travel it is about 2 weeks later. Always wear a seatbelt; injuries in automobile accidents tend to be less serious when you are buckled up.

Alternative hint

Natural, nonmedical methods of pain relief during delivery entail: relaxation and quiet breathing; water (warm bath or shower, delivery bath); firm lower-back massage; sitting upright (lean forward slightly ~ contractions are less painful, but more effective) and emotional support.

Practical hint

Ask your doctor what pain relief options are available during delivery and discuss the best ones for *you*. Some examples are Demerol, epidural block or spinal block.

Medical hint

Danger signals: severe headache, blurred vision, abdominal pain, vaginal bleeding, leaking amniotic fluid, reduced movements by the baby ~ call doctor or go to hospital immediately.

Lower back massage

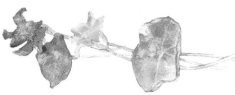

monday

tuesday

wednesday

thursday

friday

saturday

sunday

n   o   t   e   s

weight   : _____
diet   : _____
exercise   : _____
habits   : _____
next doctor's appointment: _____/_____/_____ at _____

- May feel short of breath.
- Stomach feels full due to growing uterus pressing against it.
- Normally feels physically fairly comfortable despite this.

Mother

- Can feel pain, is alarmed by loud noises.
- Length: 16 inches (40cm); weight: 3lb (1.4kg).

Baby

Lifestyle

Eat smaller meals more frequently.

To prevent heartburn at night, limit liquid intake after evening meal.

Alternative hint

Experiment with different positions for delivery ~ the more upright and mobile you are, the quicker the delivery will be.

Other positions:

- Sit on low chair and hold on to partner (supported squatting position).
- Kneel or stand and lean forward, holding onto arm of chair for support.
- Stand on hands and knees (all fours).

Practical hint

It may be necessary for the working woman to adapt her workload ~ pain is always a warning signal.

Medical hint

Braxton-Hicks contractions are uncomfortable, but not painful. They now become more regular in preparation of birth.

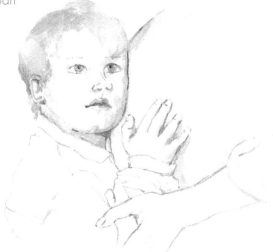

Feel baby kicking

Rosemary

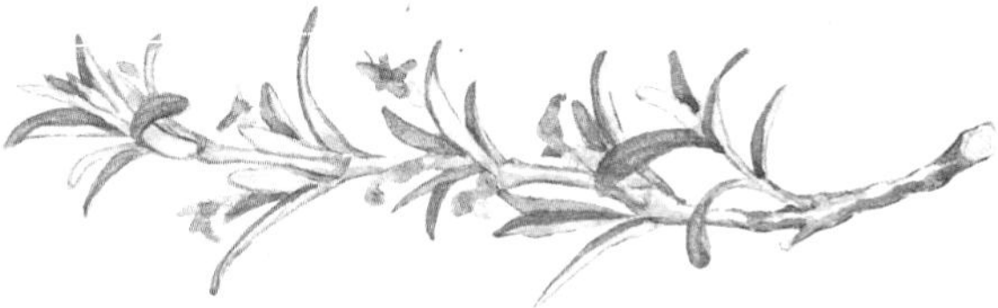

monday

tuesday

wednesday

thursday

friday

saturday

sunday

n o t e s

weight : ________

diet : ____

exercise : ____

habits : ____

next doctor's appointment: _____/_____/_____ at __________

- May leak drops of urine when laughing or coughing.
- Navel pressed flat ~ may even start protruding.
- Pelvic discomfort due to pressure and stress on joints.

Mother

Baby

- Usually lies with head down.
- In boys, the testes move down into the scrotum.
- Length: 16.2 inches (40.5cm); weight: 3.5lb (1.6kg).

Lifestyle

Rest regularly during the day and put feet up if possible.
Keep up the pelvic-floor exercises.

Alternative hint

20% of pregnant women experience numbness or pain in hands, particularly at night (carpal tunnel syndrome) ~ massaging and stretching exercises for the wrists, or splints at night, may provide relief.

Practical hint

If your other child(ren) is small, a surprise gift from the new baby is a good idea.
Get it ready to take along to the hospital or clinic.

Medical hint

Should the baby be born now, it has a 90% chance of survival.
An ultrasound examination to evaluate blood flow to, and growth of, baby is invaluable now.

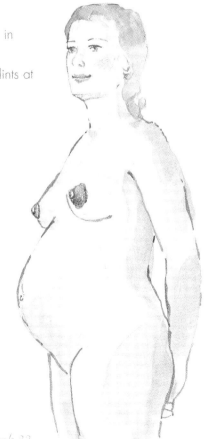

monday

tuesday

wednesday

thursday

friday

saturday

sunday

n   o   t   e   s

weight   : _____
diet   : _____
exercise   : _____
habits   : _____
next doctor's appointment: _____/_____/_____ at _____

- Sleep is often restless.
- Often dreams of abnormal baby and/or traumatic delivery (this is *not* an omen!)

Mother

Baby

- Skin smoother and less wrinkled.
- Fingernails fully formed, toenails not.
- *Vernix caseosa* (waxy substance covering fetal skin) thicker.
- Length: 16.5 inches (41.5cm); weight: 4lb (1.8kg).

Lifestyle

To grandparents, the arrival of a grandchild is a precious experience ~ take special care to include them in the pregnancy.

Alternative hint

Insomnia (aggravated by tension, indigestion, discomfort, bladder problems, cramps, etc.):

- Avoid food or stimulants (tea or coffee) before bedtime.
- Chamomile or limeflower tea may help.
- Calcium and magnesium supplements (or a glass of milk) before bedtime may help.
- Extra pillows may help.

Practical hint

Rinse all the baby's clothes and blankets. Make sure everything is ready for baby's arrival.

Medical hint

Diabetes in the mother is dangerous to the baby; ensure that blood sugar is controlled. Mothers with multiple pregnancies, such as twins, or triplets, often have early deliveries ~ prenatal care is very important.

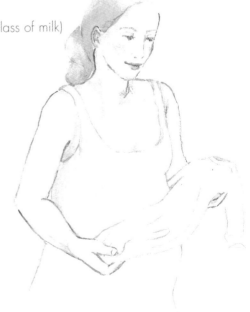

Clothes inspection

monday

....
....
....

tuesday

....
....

wednesday

....
....
....

thursday

....
....

friday

....
....
....

saturday

....
....

sunday

....
....
....

n o t e s

weight   : _____
diet   : _____
exercise   : _____
habits   : _____
next doctor's appointment: _____/_____/_____ at _____

week 34

- Underside of rib cage may be painful due to pressure of uterus and kicking of the baby.
- Urination frequency increases.
- Sleeping problems are common.

Mother

Baby

- Fingernails reach fingertips.
- Eyes blink.
- Lungs almost mature.
- Baby usually lying in position for delivery by now.
- Length: 17.2 inches (43cm); weight: 4.5lb (2kg).

Lifestyle

Take special care to look good and dress with style.
Have your hair cut in a convenient style for after the birth.
Do not wear tight-fitting clothes!

Alternative hint

If you prefer a home delivery, make all the necessary preparations. A midwife should provide the necessary instructions. Black plastic garbage bags under the sheets will prevent blood stains on the mattress. String and a sterile pair of scissors are needed for cutting the umbilical cord. Arrange for medical assistance in case of an emergency.

Practical hint

Put all the requirements for changing baby's diaper in one container (cotton balls or washcloth, ointment, rubbing alcohol for care of the umbilical cord ~ and diapers).

Medical hint

If the baby is lying with its buttocks downward (breech position), the doctor can now try to turn the baby.

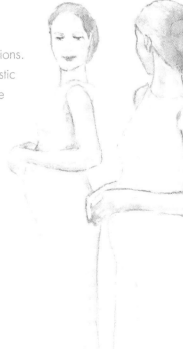

monday

tuesday

wednesday

thursday

friday

saturday

sunday

n   o   t   e   s

weight   : _____
diet   : _____
exercise   : _____
habits   : _____
next doctor's appointment: _____/_____/_____ at _____

- Feels tired and emotional.
- Urinates often due to pressure on the bladder.
- Sleeping problems may continue.

Mother

Baby

- Movements suppressed due to limited space, but still active.
- Length: 17.8 inches (44.5cm); weight: 5lb (2.3kg).

Lifestyle

Take sufficient calcium ~ baby takes precedence and will use the mother's reserves if necessary (this may lead to osteoporosis later on).
1,200mg calcium required daily (also during breastfeeding) ~ dairy products, broccoli and sardines are good sources.

Practical hints

Obtain a list of requirements for the hospital and pack your bag:
For hospital: • T-shirt for delivery + 3 nightdresses (pajamas that open in front are convenient for breastfeeding); • massage oil; • camera; • hairbrush, elastic band for hair; • 2 washcloths; • gown, slippers; • toothbrush and toothpaste; • snacks, fruit juices; • laundry bag; • nursing bra and pads, panties, sanitary napkins.
For homecoming: • loose-fitting clothes for mother; • for baby: bib, "onesies", booties, blanket, infant car seat, 2 disposable diapers.

Medical hint

Birth is divided into 3 stages:
Stage 1: Contractions open cervix (mouth of uterus) from 0 to 10 cm (active labor only starts at 3cm; thereafter it proceeds at 1cm an hour on average).
Stage 2: Birth of baby ~ could take up to 60 minutes.
Stage 3: Release of placenta (afterbirth).

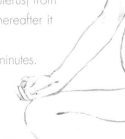

Meditation

monday

tuesday

wednesday

thursday

friday

saturday

sunday

n o t e s

weight : _____
diet : _____
exercise : _____
habits : _____
next doctor's appointment: _____/_____/_____ at _____

week 36

Mother

- Uterus reaches highest point at bottom of breastbone.
- Very uncomfortable (also because of 12 to 15kg weight gain).
- Concerns about labor and delivery are normal.

- Baby gains about an ounce a day.
- Still actively moving around.
- Length: 18.5 inches (46cm); weight: 5.5lb (2.5kg).

Baby

Lifestyle

Pamper yourself and pay special attention to your partner. Appreciate him and make time to see to his needs. Consider him and spoil him ~ with his favorite meal, tickets to a movie or a surprise gift.

Alternative hint

Spoil yourself ~ with facials, hydrotherapy, a massage and hair treatments.

Practical hint

Make arrangements for your other child(ren) during the birth, including assistance with ride clubs, etc., during your first few days back at home. Buy nursing bras (at least 2). Register at the hospital (if not done yet). Prepare food for after the birth (cook double portions and freeze half).

Medical hint

Emergency delivery: Keep calm and send for help. This is a natural event ~ wrap the baby in a clean towel or blanket and tie off the umbilical cord with 2 pieces of string (about 4 inches or 10cm apart, and about 6 and 10 inches (15 and 25cm) from the baby) and cut it off between the strings. Placenta can be removed at the hospital or clinic.

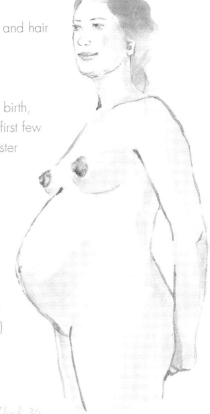

monday

tuesday

wednesday

thursday

friday

saturday

sunday

n   o   t   e   s

weight   : _____
diet   : _____
exercise   : _____
habits   : _____
next doctor's appointment: _____/_____/_____ at _____

Mother

- Feels better as soon as the baby starts moving into the pelvis.
- Pressure in pelvis, rectum and bladder.
- Stitch in the leg (pressure on nerve) is common.

- Strong movement despite the limited space.
- Amniotic fluid starts reducing.
- Lungs more mature.
- Head starts moving into the pelvis in first pregnancy.
- Length: 18.8 inches (47cm); weight: 6lb (2.7kg).

Baby

Lifestyle

Approach delivery in a positive way ~ be well-informed.
Good communication with doctor or midwife is essential.
Do not go on any long trips.

Alternative hint

Keep alternative birth plan in mind ~ everything does not always go according to plan. A Cesarean section is a major operation ~ be informed about it. Do not consider yourself a failure if the delivery does not go according to plan ~ life often takes its own course!

Practical hint

Visit the hospital and maternity ward. Check visiting hours and regulations, particularly with regard to visits by your other child(ren).

Medical hint

Premature birth takes place before 37 completed weeks. Multiple pregnancies (twins, triplets) often go into labor earlier. *Warning:* Stomachache coupled with bleeding or vaginal discharge must be reported to the doctor immediately.

Massage

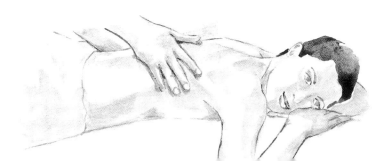

monday

tuesday

wednesday

thursday

friday

saturday

sunday

n o t e s

weight : _____
diet : _____
exercise : _____
habits : _____
next doctor's appointment: _____/_____/_____ at _____

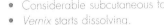

week 38

- Impatient, tired of waiting.
- Baby does not necessarily drop into the pelvis. (This is more often seen in first pregnancy.)

Mother

Baby

- Considerable subcutaneous fat.
- *Vernix* starts dissolving.
- Length: 19.2 inches (48cm); weight: 6.4lb (2.9kg).

Lifestyle

Be patient, relax and try to enjoy the last few days.

Alternative hint

Acupuncture and hypnosis may provide pain control, as may aromatherapy, massage and reflexology, if applied correctly.

Practical hint

Decide on pain relief options you want to use, previously discussed with your doctor.

Medical hint

Signs of delivery: Regular painful contractions; "show" (mucus plug from the cervix, often with bleeding); amniotic fluid drains ("waters breaking"); bleeding.
Contact doctor or midwife immediately.
99% of babies are normal at birth. 85% of births are without intervention; that is, without complications.

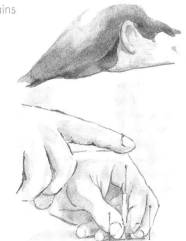

Acupuncture

monday

tuesday

wednesday

thursday

friday

saturday

sunday

n o t e s

weight : _____
diet : _____
exercise : _____
habits : _____
next doctor's appointment: _____/_____/_____ at _____

week 39

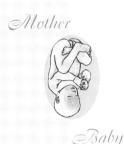

- Braxton-Hicks contractions become stronger and more regular.
- May lose weight.

Mother

Baby

- Still fed by placenta, but can function independently.
- Movements now much less because of limited space.
- Length: 19.6 inches (49cm); weight: 6.8lb (3.1kg).

Lifestyle

Relax and save energy for birth. There will be time after the birth of the baby to finish household chores (do not try to do too much now).

Alternative hint

Reflexology is a system in which the foot, and sometimes the hand, is massaged in specific places to affect other parts of the body therapeutically. It can be used both for relaxation and to induce labor naturally, among other uses. Look for books on this topic at your library or schedule an appointment with a reflexologist if you are interested.

Practical hint

Keep list of emergency telephone numbers on hand. Make a list of names and telephone numbers of people to inform after the birth.

Medical hint

Breech delivery: about 4% of babies are born buttocks first. Very good cooperation is required from the mother for a normal birth; in first pregnancies, this position mostly results in a Cesarean birth.

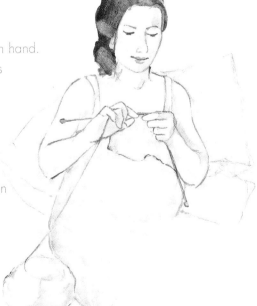

Relaxing

monday

tuesday

wednesday

thursday

friday

saturday

sunday

n   o   t   e   s

weight   : _____
diet   : _____
exercise   : _____
habits   : _____
next doctor's appointment: _____/_____/_____ at _____

week 40

- Only 5% of babies are born on the due date, so be patient. Most babies are born in the 2 weeks on either side of the due date.

Mother

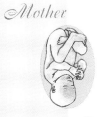

Baby

- About 20oz (600ml) urine produced a day.
- *Vernix* covering reduces further.
- Lies relatively still while waiting to be born.
- Length: 20 inches (50cm); weight: 5.5 to 7.5lb (2.5 to 3.5 kg).

Lifestyle

Keep yourself occupied ~ time will pass more quickly.

Sleep on your side with a pillow propped between your thighs.

Alternative hint

Approach the delivery positively and stay in control of the situation. Familiarize yourself with the stages of delivery; realize that birth pains *are* painful, but they pass quickly (the strongest contractions last about 1 minute and occur 3 to 4 times every 10 minutes). Use the time between contractions to relax and focus on the main aim: The birth of a healthy baby makes all pain and suffering fade away.

Practical hint

Do not be disappointed if there is a change in the birth plan ~ the ideal is the safe delivery of a healthy baby to a healthy mother. You could not hope for a more positive experience than that!

Medical hint

"Show" (mucus plug in the cervix, often with bleeding), drainage and "waters breaking" (leaking of amniotic fluid) and regular, painful contractions indicate start of labor.

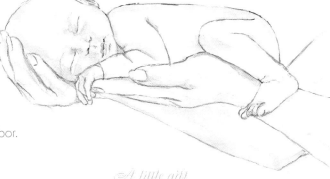

A little gift

week 41

monday

tuesday

wednesday

thursday

friday

saturday

sunday

week 42

monday

tuesday

wednesday

thursday

friday

saturday

sunday

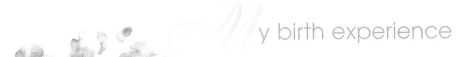

My birth experience

First impressions of baby

after the
Birth

The birth of a baby radically changes the lives of the new mother and father, but it is one of the most enriching experiences imaginable. The unconditional love of a small child makes life that much more worthwhile. No book or advice can, however, prepare you fully for the adjustments a newborn baby demands from the mother and family.

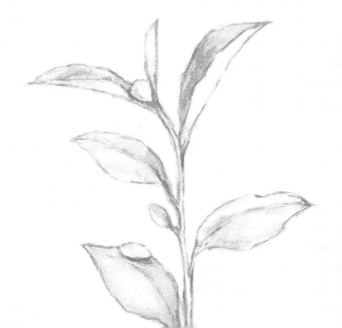

Violet

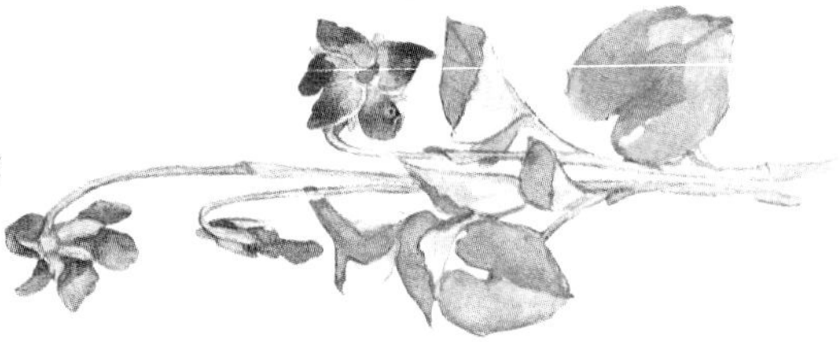

monday

tuesday

wednesday

thursday

friday

saturday

sunday

n o t e s

weight : ______

diet : ______

exercise : ______

habits : ______

next doctor's appointment: ____/____/____ at ______

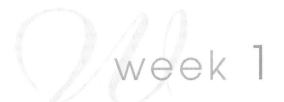

Mother

- Colostrum is produced only by day 3 or 4 ("the milk comes in"). Breasts full and painful.
- Episiotomy or lacerations painful.
- Abdominal wall often flabby.
- Vaginal discharge (*lochia*) bloody at first; becomes paler and disappears after a few weeks.
- Day 3: "baby blues" ~ 80% of women.

Baby

- Head misshapen (after vaginal delivery), eyes swollen, vernix in skin wrinkles, body covered with fine down. • Sense of touch well developed. • Sleeps 70 to 80% of day; feeds approximately 7 times a day; reacts to sounds; focuses up to 12 inches (30cm). • Recognizes mother's voice and smell from day one.

Lifestyle

After Cesarean section: Start moving as soon as possible (it makes the pain more bearable). Breastfeeding is an acquired skill; obtain help, if necessary.

Alternative hint

Ice pack between legs immediately after delivery reduces swelling and pain. Disinfect vaginal lacerations or episiotomy wound with saline sitz bath 3 times a day (approximately half an ounce [15ml] coarse salt dissolved in a shallow bath or basin of lukewarm water).

Medical hint

Congested breasts: Let the baby drink regularly; rub painful, hard lumps in the breasts while baby is drinking and express milk if necessary. Milk production takes place according to demand; regular feeding improves milk production. Do not let baby suckle for too long initially (approximately 5 minutes) and interrupt sucking (press down onto chin or put little finger into mouth) before taking baby off the breast. This prevents sore, bleeding nipples. Postnatal pains can be severe ~ take painkillers from day 2 for a few days. These painful contractions of the uterus occur during breastfeeding.

Mother's milk

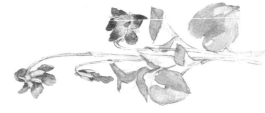

monday

_____
_____
_____

tuesday

_____
_____
_____

wednesday

_____
_____
_____

thursday

_____
_____
_____

friday

_____
_____
_____

saturday

_____
_____
_____

sunday

_____
_____
_____

n   o   t   e   s

weight   : _____
diet   : _____
exercise   : _____
habits   : _____
next doctor's appointment: _____/_____/_____ at _____

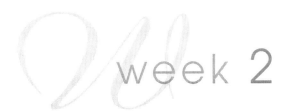

- *Breast congestion (engorgement):* Express milk; feed less regularly and place cabbage leaves on breasts to relieve swelling.
- Need not feel overwhelming love for baby ~ it could take weeks for mother and baby bonding to take place.

Mother

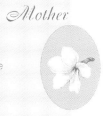

Baby

- Prefers patterns (curves, spirals, checks) with high contrast (black and white). • Hearing, smell and taste well developed.
- Reaches birth weight again on approximately day 7 to 10.
- Umbilical cord shrinks and falls off from day 7 to 14 (or earlier).

Lifestyle

Expect to wear loose-fitting clothes for another few weeks. Start doing some gentle exercises, particularly for the stomach muscle and pelvic floor.

Alternative hint

Rest while the baby is sleeping. Practice relaxation techniques.

Practical hint

Apply for baby's social security number.

Bathe baby in a warm room. It is unnecessary to bathe the baby completely and wash his or her hair every day.

Never leave baby alone in the bath. A rubber mat or washcloth in the bath will prevent baby from slipping when soaped.

Medical hint

Danger signals in newborn baby: Seizures; labored breathing; abnormal sleepiness; abnormal crying; refusing food for 1 day; vomiting and diarrhea; redness of skin around the navel. Consult doctor or nurse.

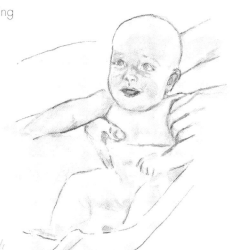

Baby bath

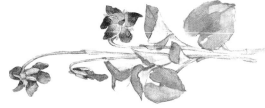

monday

tuesday

wednesday

thursday

friday

saturday

sunday

n o t e s

weight : _____
diet : _____
exercise : _____
habits : _____
next doctor's appointment: _____/_____/_____ at _____

- Get as much rest as possible ~ it takes 6 weeks to regain your strength.
- The birth of a baby often strengthens the bond between the new mother and her own mother.

Mother

Baby

- Demand feeding is ideal with preferably fewer regular night feeds. Never try to feed more than every 2 hours (preferably every 3 to 4 hours).
- Always support the neck when picking up baby.
- Still sleeps most of the time.

Lifestyle

Try to get baby into a routine. Carefully introduce baby to pets.
During breastfeeding: Drink 8 to 12 glasses of water each day.
Continue with pregnancy vitamin supplements; 2 glasses of milk a day provide the extra calcium required.

Alternative hint

Massaging the baby's body is very soothing. Use baby oil and rub firmly over limbs and body. Stomach cramps could also be relieved in this way.

Practical hint

Put down baby when he/she is sleepy, but not yet asleep. Do not rock to sleep ~ causes less sleeping problems later.

Medical hint

Safe to resume intercourse. Vaginal dryness is common during breastfeeding (use a water-based lubricant). Breastfeeding makes the uterus contract sooner to its pre-pregnancy size and increases energy consumption, so you regain your figure sooner. Keep 1 bottle of expressed milk on hand in case a problem arises with milk production.

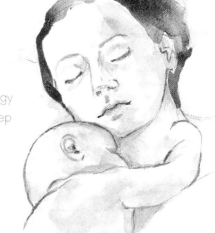

Sleeping beauties

monday

tuesday

wednesday

thursday

friday

saturday

sunday

n o t e s

weight   : _____
diet   : _____
exercise   : _____
habits   : _____
next doctor's appointment: _____/_____/_____ at _____

Mother

- Postnatal depression occurs in 20% of women. Usually starts between 4 weeks and 3 months after the birth. It is serious ~ medical and psychological help is required urgently.
- Loses interest in virtually everything, has difficulty in making simple decisions and doing daily chores.

Baby

- Smiles broadly with twinkling eyes.
- Still sleeps for long stretches, but waking hours now longer.

Lifestyle

The father has to adjust to receiving less attention (temporarily) and experiences more financial stress. Make special time for him ~ listen to what he says and be sensitive to his needs.

Alternative hints

Always handle baby calmly.
Never try to quiet baby by shaking it ~ this can cause baby serious harm.

Practical hint

Do not keep mixed formula milk out of the refrigerator for longer than 1 hour ~ carry powder and cooled boiled water separately when traveling.

Medical hint

Consult doctor or clinic if experiencing any of the following: Unpleasant vaginal discharge; tender abdomen; fever; severe vaginal bleeding; extremely painful episiotomy wound; swollen and painful calf muscles.

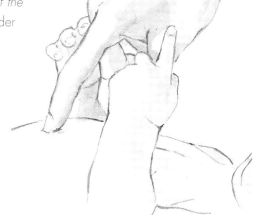

Touch baby gently

monday

tuesday

wednesday

thursday

friday

saturday

sunday

n o t e s

weight   : _____
diet   : _____
exercise   : _____
habits   : _____
next doctor's appointment: _____/_____/_____ at _____

- Breastfeeding established ~ produces an average of 30oz (850ml) breast milk a day.
- Vaginal discharge (*lochia*) should disappear.
- Becoming a mother can be exhausting, so get as much rest as you can.

Mother

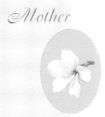

- Improved neck control.
- Improved sleeping and feeding routine.

Baby

Lifestyle

Integrate baby into the family. Involve grandparents in handling and care of their new grandchild. Just as it is a privilege for grandma and grandpa to have grandchildren, so it is a privilege for the grandchild to know its grandparents.

Alternative hint

Mother is entitled to time on her own for relaxation and emotional recovery. Motherhood is an immense adjustment. Lack of sleep and exhaustion often cause the new mother to become unsure of her capabilities. The emotional adjustment develops with time.

Practical hint

Do not allow people to smoke near the baby.

Medical hint

Babies cry for attention ~ when tired, ill, hungry or diaper is wet. Initially it is difficult to know how to react correctly. Ensure that baby is comfortable, has had enough to drink and been burped, and handle calmly.

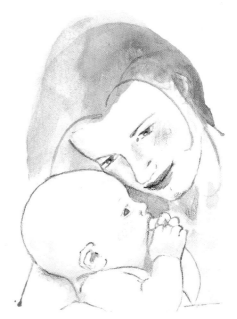

Mother and child

monday

tuesday

wednesday

thursday

friday

saturday

sunday

n o t e s

weight : _____
diet : _____
exercise : _____
habits : _____
next doctor's appointment: _____/_____/_____ at _____

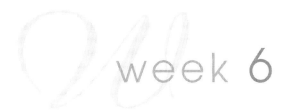

Mother

- Uterus back to pre-pregnancy size.
- Varicose veins and hemorrhoids improved.
- Resumption of menstruation:
  If bottle-feeding: menstruation starts 4 to 6 weeks after delivery.
  If breastfeeding: menstruation could be absent for months.

Baby

- Follows moving objects with eyes.
- Reacts to voices.
- Prefers bright primary colors, as well as the contrast between black and white.
- Is alarmed by sudden noises.

Lifestyle

If the mother is happy and relaxed, the baby will also be happy and content. Children of parents who laugh often, also laugh more often.

Alternative hint

Not having baby immunized is strongly discouraged.

Practical hint

Visit to the doctor by mother and baby: Baby must visit clinic for immunization.

Medical hint

You can become fertile within 6 weeks after birth. It is therefore important to practice birth control if you do not want to become pregnant right away.
Contraception (birth control):

- Progestogen pill (mini-pill) or injection.
- Sterilization after giving birth.
- Intrauterine device 6 weeks after birth.

Baby's growth and development evaluated for the first time at the 6-week examination. Reflexes and hips, heart, lungs and bowels also evaluated.

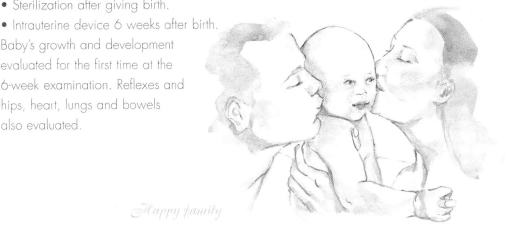

Happy family

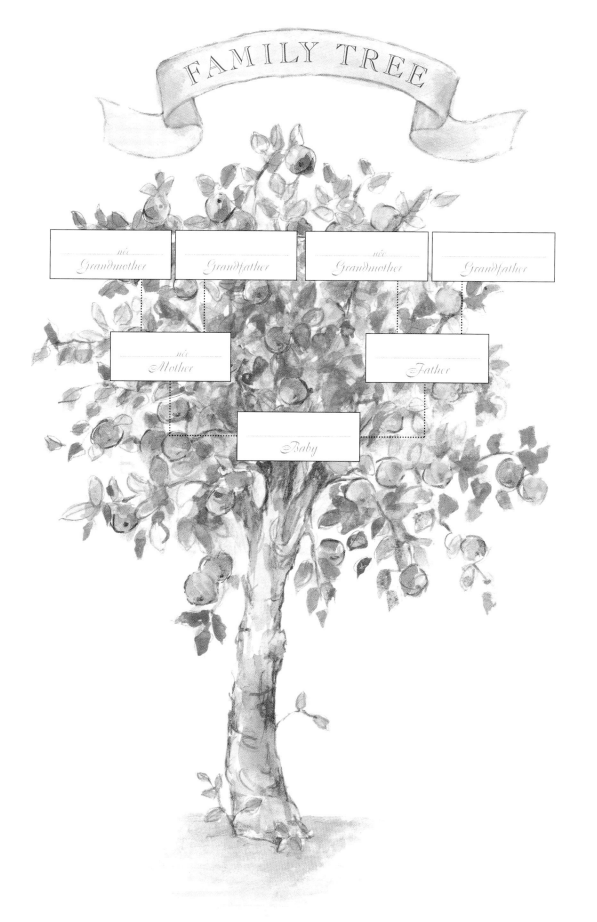

FAMILY TREE

_____ née _____
Grandmother

Grandfather

_____ née _____
Grandmother

Grandfather

_____ née _____
Mother

Father

Baby

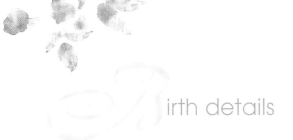

Birth details

Name:

Place:

Date:

Time:

Sex:

Weight:

Length:

Doctor:

Other:

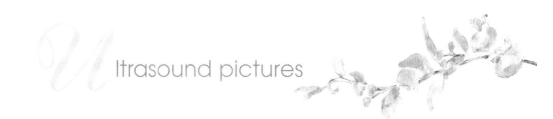

Ultrasound pictures

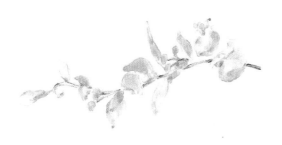

Photographs

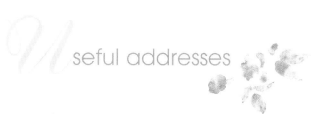

Useful addresses

Accident prevention

SafetyBeltSafe
P.O. Box 553
Altadena, CA 91003
(800) 745-SAFE

The Danny Foundation
(information on crib dangers)
3158 Danville Blvd.
Alamo, CA 94507
(800) 83-DANNY

U.S. Consumer Product Safety
Commission Hotline
(800) 638-2772

Breastfeeding

INFACT Canada
10 Trinity Square
Toronto, Ont. M5G 1B1
(416) 595-9819

La Leche League International
1400 N. Meacham Rd.
Schaumburg, IL 60173
(847) 519-7730; (800) LA-LECHE

Medela, Inc.
P.O. Box 660
McHenry, IL 60051
(800) TELL-YOU
Information, referral for breast pumps, breastfeeding
specialists

Medical Information

American College of Obstetricians
and Gynecologists (ACOG)
Resource Center
P.O. Box 96920
Washington, DC 20090-6920
Information about pregnancy, labor, birth or
postpartum issues. Include SASE.

Family Service Canada
600-220 Laurier Ave.
West Ottawa, Ont. K1P 5Z9
(613) 230-9960

National Center for Nutrition and Dietetics'
Consumer Nutrition Hotline
(to talk directly with a nutritionist)
(800) 366-1655

Help for Mother

American Cancer Society
Help to quit smoking; check phone book for
local affiliate.
(800) 227-2345

Childbirth Options

American Society for Psychoprophylaxis in Obstetrics
(ASPO/Lamaze)
1200 19 Street NW
Suite 300
Washington, DC 20036-2422
(800) 368-4404

Doulas of North America
1100 23rd Ave. East
Seattle, WA 98112
Fax: (206) 325-0472
www.dona.com

Informed Home Birth
(313) 662-6857

International Cesarean Awareness Network (ICAN)
1304 Kingsdale Rd.
Redondo Beach, CA 90278
(310) 542-6400

Midwives Alliance of North America (MANA)
P.O. Box 175
Newton, KS 57115
(612) 854-8660

Multiples

National Organization of Mothers of
Twins Clubs, Inc.
P.O. Box 23188
Albuquerque, NM 87102-1188
(800) 243-2276
www.nomotc.org

Triplet Connection
P.O. Box 99571
Stockton, CA 95209
(209) 474-0885

Postnatal Depression

Depression after Delivery
P.O. Box 1282
Morrisville, PA 19067
(800) 944-4773 (answering machine)

Sudden Infant Death Syndrome

(SIDS)
National SIDS Alliance
1314 Bedford Ave.
Suite 210
Baltimore, MD 21208
(800) 221-SIDS
Fax: (410) 964-8009

Crisis Help

National Child Abuse Hotline
(for parents in crisis or children at risk)
(800) 4A-CHILD (800-422-4453)